What Does the Bible Say About Us?

What Does the Bible Say,
and Why Should I Care?

What's in the Bible About Us?

Alex Joyner

ABINGDON PRESS
NASHVILLE

WHAT'S IN THE BIBLE ABOUT US?
by Alex Joyner

Copyright © 2008 by Abingdon Press

All rights reserved. No part of this work may be reproduced or transmitted in any form or by any means, electronic or mechanical, including photocopying and recording, or by any information or retrieval system, except as may be expressly permitted in the 1976 Copyright Act or in writing from the publisher. Requests for permission should be addressed in writing to Permissions Office, P. O. Box 801, 201 Eighth Avenue, South, Nashville, Tennessee 37202-0801, or call (615) 749-6421.

Scripture quotations in this publication unless otherwise indicated, are from the New Revised Standard Version of the Bible, copyright © 1989 by the Division of Christian Education of the National Council of the Churches of Christ in the United States of America, and are used by permission. All rights reserved.

Abingdon Press

ISBN-13: 978-0-687-65373-7

Manufactured in the United States of America

08 09 10 11 12 13 14 15 16 17—10 9 8 7 6 5 4 3 2 1

CONTENTS

About the Writer vi
A Word From the Editor vii
A Word From the Writer ix
1. God Created Us 1
2. God Cares for Us 21
3. God Saves Us 39
4. God Invites Us Into Relationship 61
Appendix: Praying the Bible 81

ABOUT THE WRITER

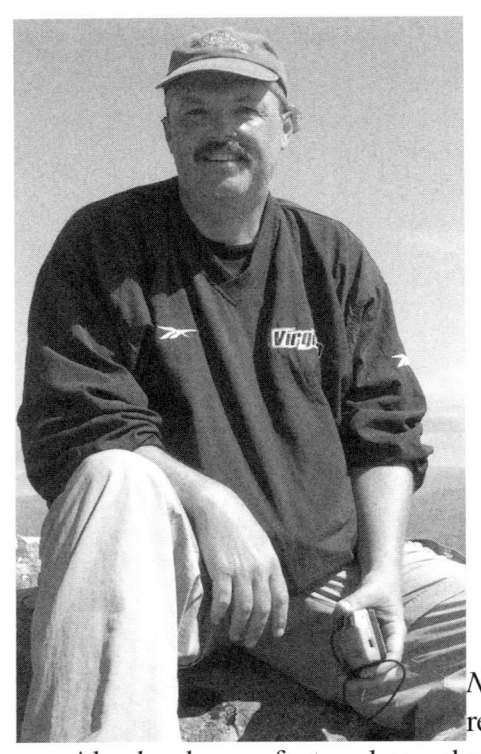

Alex Joyner is a United Methodist pastor serving on the Eastern Shore of Virginia, one of the last undeveloped coastal regions on the Eastern seaboard. Alex serves Franktown Church, a vibrant congregation representing the diversity of the region. In previous roles, he has worked in inner-city Dallas, Texas, as a youth director; as an associate pastor in a bilingual Latino congregation; as a pastor in England and Virginia; and as a campus minister at the University of Virginia. His experience with college students and young adults led him to write *Restless Hearts: Where Do I Go Now, God?* (Abingdon Press), a resource for discovering your vocation.

Alex has been a featured preacher on the former *Protestant Hour* radio broadcast (now *Day One*) and began his career as a radio news director. He is summer adjunct lecturer at Southern Methodist University, where he has taught Bible and theology courses since 1996. He has a great interest in missions and has led work teams domestically and in Mexico. He has also led a student group to two places of Christian pilgrimage—Taize, France, and Iona, Scotland. Alex is an avid kayaker who is often found paddling in the marshes and bays near his home. He is married to Suzanne and has two children, Joel and Rachel.

A WORD FROM THE EDITOR

About This Bible Study Series

Have you ever wondered what the Bible is all about? What's in it? Why is it so important for Christians? Is it relevant for people in the 21st century? Should I care about what's in the Bible? Why? What difference will it make in my life? The study series *What's in the Bible, and Why Should I Care?* offers opportunities for you to explore these questions and others by opening the Bible, reading it, prayerfully reflecting on what the Bible readings say, and making connections between the readings and your daily life. The series title points to the two essential features of meaningful Bible study: reading the Bible and applying it to your life. This unique and exciting Bible study series is designed to help you accomplish this two-fold purpose.

The books in *What's in the Bible, and Why Should I Care?* are designed to help you find relevance, hope, and meaning for your life even if you have little or no experience with the Bible. You will discover ways the Bible can help you with major questions you may have about the nature of God, how God relates to us, and how we can relate to God. Such questions continue to be relevant whether you are new to church life, a longtime member of church, or a seeker who is curious and wants to know more.

Whether you read a study book from this series on your own or with others in a Bible study group, you will experience benefits. You will gain confidence in reading the Bible as you learn how to use and study it. You will find meaning and hope in the people and teachings of the Bible. Most important of all, you will discover more about who God is and how God relates to you personally through the Bible.

What's in the Bible?

Obviously, we answer the question "What's in the Bible?" by reading it. As Christians, we understand that the stories of our faith come to us through this holy book. We view the Bible as the central document for all we believe and profess about God. It contains stories about those who came

A WORD FROM THE EDITOR

before us in the Christian faith, but it is more than a book of stories about them. The Bible tells us about God. It tells how a particular group of people in a particular part of the world over an extended period of time, inspired by God, understood and wrote about who God is and how God acted among them. It also tells what God expected from them. Its value and meaning reach to all people across all time—past, present, and future.

Why Should I Care?

Meaningful Bible study inspires people to live their lives according to God's will and way. As you read through the stories collected in the Bible, you will see again and again a just and merciful God who creates, loves, saves, and heals. You will see that God expects people, who are created in the image of God (Genesis 1), to live their lives as just and merciful people of God. You will discover that God empowers people to live according to God's way. You will learn that in spite of our sin, of our tendency to turn away from God and God's ways, God continues to love and save us. This theme emerges from and unifies all the books that have been brought together in the Holy Bible.

Christians believe that God's work of love and salvation finds confirmation and completion through the life, ministry, death, and resurrection of Jesus Christ. We accept God's free gift of love and salvation through Jesus Christ; and out of gratitude, we commit our lives to following him and living as he taught us to live. Empowered by God's Holy Spirit, we grow in faith, service, and love toward God and neighbor. I pray that this Bible study series will help you experience God's love and power in your daily life. I pray that it will help you grow in your faith and commitment to Jesus Christ.

Pamela Dilmore

A WORD FROM THE WRITER

I won't forget the day that I realized I was an adult. It was a bit of a disappointment. I was in my late twenties and leading a congregation as its pastor. In that role I was confronting things each day that made me question my qualifications for the job. What do you say in the face of death? For that matter, how do you give expression to the meaning of a birth? I sometimes thought of what I was doing as filling the place of pastor until the real adult showed up. Then one day I realized something startling: I was the adult I had been waiting for. I would still have elders and contemporaries that I could rely on for wisdom; but however I felt about myself, others would see me as a fully formed adult.

In truth, we are never fully formed. One of the amazing things about being human is that we are always on a journey of self-understanding. Throughout our lives we will find ourselves wondering at how the world looks from a new vantage point. New relationships, a health crisis, parenthood, losing a job, overcoming an addiction, losing a loved one—all of these moments can significantly alter our sense of self; but if we are open to it, these can also be moments of growth.

So why look to the Bible for information about who we are as human beings and as individuals? It is a strange book, after all. How can a collection of stories and writings from communities that are now long since gone have anything to say to 21st-century people?

The Bible remains a powerful voice in the world, especially among Christian people, for the very reason that it can give us ourselves. Generations have been formed by these stories and have listened for God in the midst of them. They have not been disappointed. Despite its strangeness—maybe because of its strangeness—the Bible has helped people to hear something about themselves that they can't hear in other places. This book is an invitation to you to take a journey into the world of the Bible and to listen for what it may say about who we are and more particularly who you are.

In the first chapter we will consider what it means to be created by God and what it means to bear the image of our Maker. The second chapter

A WORD FROM THE WRITER

explores the nature of God's care for human beings and wonders aloud at how vulnerable and often flawed creatures retain that love. The third chapter introduces the biblical notion of salvation and looks at the varied ways the Bible talks about God's saving work. In the final chapter we look at what it means to be in relationship to God and how that affects our identity.

We should begin with a word of explanation. Even though I will often talk about what the Bible says, you should hear something else in that. The Bible is the product of centuries of voices giving witness to who God is and who we are. Some of those voices are powerful speaking from the perspective of those who experienced success and influence in life. Some of those voices speak from the underside where the word of God comes into a world of suffering and marginalization. So even though we will talk about the Bible as if it is one voice with a single story to tell, behind the Bible is a community of the faithful who have seen the myriad ways that human beings live and act. What makes the Bible a rich resource is the way that it lets those many experiences of humanity shine through.

Who am I to tell this story? I have been ordained for almost 20 years now. I have worked in cross-cultural settings in Texas, Virginia, and England. I have walked with college students as a campus minister. I have taught theology and Bible to other ministers. I am a husband and the father of two amazing children. None of these qualifies me to answer the question posed by the title of this book, though. My greatest qualification, I believe, is that I am human and still wondering what that means. At times it feels like that should be the easiest thing in the world to answer. When I am at home in my own skin, it doesn't pose any difficulties; but when I consider the wonder and complexity of human life and my own soul, I know that there are many things yet to understand. The Bible has been my companion for many years in this journey. It is still an essential guidebook.

So whether you have some history with the Bible or whether you are coming to it for the first time, I hope that you will find in this book an introduction to a deeper life with the God whose story we will encounter here. The writer of the First Letter of John offered this affirmation to one

A WORD FROM THE WRITER

of those early Christian communities: "Beloved, we are God's children now; what we will be has not yet been revealed" (1 John 3:2). I offer the same affirmation here. We may not yet be fully formed adults, and we await the revelation of who we will be; but there is the assurance that we can be God's children now.

I give thanks for the opportunity to think out loud with you about these most basic questions. I thank as well my usual partners in my journey for their insight and wisdom. From students to teachers to family to congregants to friends and fellow travelers, I have come to know this truth: that the world is fierce and vast and devastating and beautiful, and God is everywhere within.

Alex Joyner

Chapter One

God Created Us

Bible Readings
Genesis 1–2; Psalm 139; John 1:1-5; Acts 17:23-28; Colossians 1:14-17

The Questions
The Christian faith teaches that humans were created by God. What does the Bible say about human beings as God's creation? How does the knowledge that we are created by God affect our understanding of ourselves? of other human beings? Take a moment and write responses to the questions.

A Psalm

> When I look at your heavens, the work of your fingers,
>> the moon and the stars that you have established;
> what are human beings that you are mindful of them,
>> mortals that you care for them?
>>> Psalm 8:3-4

A Prayer

God, you are beyond words. You are beyond the capacity of my mind to understand, but I trust that you can enlighten me. You are beyond all things, but I believe that you are here. Remind me who I am. Speak through and beyond these words; but most of all, speak in me; in Christ's name. Amen.

Listening for God

In order to talk about what it means to be created by God, the best place to start is probably with a time when you could not talk. What did you describe? Was it when you received a great gift you were not expecting? Maybe it was at the birth of a child. Perhaps it was when you took a hike on a trail and turned a corner to see a marsh or a mountain that was impossibly beautiful—the kind of scene for which the word *inexpressible* was invented. Or was it in the midst of an argument when you were suddenly confronted with another dimension of the person in front of you that you had never seen before? Maybe you saw something about yourself in the argument that left you without words.

> *Try to imagine the last time that you were speechless. Describe the circumstances. Who was there? What happened?*
>
> **REFLECT**

Why should you care what the Bible says about who we are as human beings? Because moments of speechlessness are rare gifts, and they are the beginning of new questions—questions people have been taking to the Bible for centuries. Before we go looking for answers, though, let's allow the Bible to help us wonder.

Try this: Find a place where you have some space to "be." Maybe it's at a table by a window with good natural light. Maybe it's that chair in the coffee shop that you know so well that you can tell someone exactly where the rip in the fabric is. Maybe it's under a tree at the park or at that spot down by the river. You know the place. Give yourself time to be with the Bible and this book.

Turn to Psalm 8. Read the whole psalm slowly, out loud if you're alone or unafraid of social consequences. Then go back to verses 3-4, which are printed at the beginning of this chapter. Ask yourself the questions. What are human beings? Who are you?

> *Read again Psalm 8:3-4. Meditate on these verses for a few minutes; and, while you do, write down words that you might use in answering these questions. What are human beings that God cares for us? Who am I?*
>
> **REFLECT**

A Story About God That Is a Story About Us

If you believe that the universe is a place best explained without resorting to words such as *mystery* and *purpose,* then the Bible will not be an easy companion. If you believe that human beings are adequately accounted for through the natural and social sciences, then the Bible will seem rather strange and unnecessary. However, if you have ever looked at the world around you, felt a deep sense of gratitude, and wondered to whom that thankfulness is due; if you have ever marveled at the ways light and shadow play in the journey of your life; if you believe that some deep meaning resides in the complexity of your relationships or that some greater truth informs your soul; if you believe that there is something holy about serving and loving others; if you are thirsting for a richer, fuller life than the ones offered in television commercials, then perhaps the Bible has a word for you.

It's part of our nature to wonder who we are. Biologists tell us that one of the things that distinguish humans from other creatures is the extended period of development that goes on after we are born. Other creatures come into the world with an instinctual self-awareness. The curse of life for a wildebeest, what it will do and how it will seek a mate, is fairly clear from the first moment. For humans such things can be influenced by a number of other factors. A duck-billed platypus is not confused about what its purpose is. It won't start a garage band or write a poem or develop a significant business partnership, but a person can.

The Chilean poet Pablo Neruda once wrote, "Whom can I ask what I came to make happen in this world?"[1] It's a question that has accompanied human beings through the ages, and it is evident throughout the pages of the Bible. This ancient text at the heart of the Christian tradition may be an account of the nature of God, but it is also a story about who we are. In the stories of the Bible we encounter men and women who find themselves as they struggle more or less successfully to be faithful to God.

The Crescendo of Creation
Genesis 1

You might think that one concern of the Bible would be to prove the existence of God, but God's existence is taken for granted in the story. Genesis 1:1, the first verse in the Bible, doesn't begin by saying, "We believe in God, and we do so for the following excellent reasons." Instead the story starts with God already in action: "In the beginning God created the heavens and the earth"[2] (New International Version). From there creation moved quickly on so that by the time the first chapter is finished we have sky, stars, sea monsters, and swarming birds among other things. God moved swiftly and with purpose. The suspense in the story is not whether there is a God, but what this God is up to. Where is this all headed?

> *What's in the Bible?*
> *Read Genesis 1. What does this Bible reading say to you about God? What does it say about the creation of the man and the woman?*

By the time we get to verse 26, it is clear what God is doing. God is capping off the world's first workweek with the creation of a man and a woman. It is not the case that all of the other days were somehow less important or that the things created before human beings were inadequate. No, in fact, God saw each day that the things created were good and delighted in the flourishing of life. However, the concert of creation did reach a crescendo with the coming of creatures made in the image of God; and there is a special role that humans play in relation to the rest of God's handiwork. God gave these humans dominion over the creatures of the sea, land, and air, indicating that they would share in the Creator's work of ordering the world (verse 28). Later, God extended this partnership to caring for the land when the first human was charged with tilling and protecting the garden of Eden (2:15).

> *The word translated as "dominion" in Genesis 1:28 is a word used of kings. What does it mean that human beings are given the role of dominion in creation? Since human beings are also given responsibility for caring for the earth, what does dominion look like? When have you felt that you were connected to the rest of creation in a way that felt like a holy partnership with God?*

Humans are created in God's image. What an astounding thing to consider! God, this great artist and lover of the universe who flings stars through the heavens, has gifted human beings with the role of partners who bear the image of the divine. It is tempting in this era, when we tally the environmental cost of human fruitfulness and multiplication (1:28), to think of humans as somehow defective and hopelessly invasive. When we look at the effect of greenhouse gas emissions, runaway land development, and intensive agriculture, we rightly believe that we should tread more gently upon the earth. We ought to learn again how to value our connectedness with the rest of the natural world; but we have not, for all of our current problems, lost what God gave us in the beginning. Being made in God's image means to be invited to join in what God is doing as co-creators.

Male and female are equal before God, both bearing the divine imprint and likeness and meant to live in a life-producing unity.

What does being created in the image of God suggest to you?

REFLECT

The Gift of Intimacy
Genesis 2

The picture of Creation given in Genesis 2 shows the depth of relationship human beings are designed to have.

What's in the Bible?
Read Genesis 2. What challenges you or makes you curious about the reading? Why? What does this Bible reading say to you about God? about human relationship?

After all the affirmations of goodness in the initial story of Creation, God declared that something was missing. Having made one human from the dust of the earth and breathing life and spirit into the human, God decided that it was not good for the human being to be alone (Genesis 2:18). When a parade of animals failed to produce a proper companion, God went back to work, sent the lone human into a deep sleep, and created a woman from a rib taken from the man's side.

The man's exclamation upon seeing the woman for the first time is one of the deepest expressions of the joy of human companionship in the Bible. "This at last," he says, "is bone of my bones and flesh of my flesh" (verse 23). The words echo God's own delight expressed in Chapter 1. You can just hear the two humans saying, "This is good. This is very good."

> *When has a close relationship helped you experience something you might call holy delight? How do our relationships help us understand who we are? When can they distract us from God?*

REFLECT

Bible Facts
The name *Adam* is closely related to the Hebrew word for the earth: *adamah*. It might be just as appropriate to talk about this first human as an earth creature rather than as a "he." The Hebrew words for a male person (*ish*) and for a female person (*ishshah*) are first used in Genesis 2:23.[3]

Does God Need Us?
Acts 17:22-28

Behind all of these pictures of who human beings are created to be lies a larger question, though. The Bible may take God's existence as a given, but why should there be human beings at all?

What's in the Bible?
Read Acts 17:22-28. How do you respond to Paul's speech to the Athenians? What words or phrases stand out for you? Why?

The grand scale of the universe suggests that it could get along quite well without us. We see our impact on the earth; but it, too, would go on, and life would continue to proliferate without humans living on the planet. God doesn't need us in order to be God either. That's not to say God doesn't care about us; it's just a statement of biblical fact.

Paul, one of the first Christian missionaries, made this same point as he talked to the philosophers on a hillside in Athens. He talked with them about a shrine to what the Athenians called "the unknown god." In essence, Paul said to them. "I know this Unknown God. This God made the world and everything in it. This God is Lord of heaven and earth and won't be contained by a shrine, even one erected in a city considered the most learned and religious in the world. This God doesn't need anything from us in order to be God."

> **Bible Facts**
> The Areopagus where Paul delivered his speech on the unknown God was the site of a court for the city of Athens in ancient Greece. The translation of the name is "Mar's Hill." Mars was the Greek god of war.

This is the wonder of creation then: God, who did not need men or women or bottlenose porpoises or redwoods or monarch butterflies or sunsets, made all these things. It is not something we can understand because we have come to know who God is through this created order. If God could get along just fine without us, why are we here?

It is hard for us to conceive of this "God who doesn't create" because the world around us tells us that it is in the very nature of God to create. It would be as easy to ask an accomplished artist why they paint or a great basketball player why they play. To experience the full joy of their gifts, the things within them have to be expressed and shared. So we might say that all the wonders, all the love, and all the potential that reside within God overflow in creation. We are the fruit of God's abundance and a source of pleasure to the God who knows that all things are good.

> *What is it that you have to do in order to be you? What is it that you have to give to the world that you can't hold in?*

Paul recognized that we are hardwired with the same tendencies as this overflowing God. The nations of the earth sprang forth from that one common ancestor, Adam; and as they became more numerous and more diverse, they used their impulse for understanding in order to seek God. The Athenians with their numerous shrines were using their art and wisdom and poetry to express their desire for the One in whom "we live and move and have our being" (Acts 17:26-28). The God Paul served has a further wonder, though. This God is great and grand and includes everything created; but this is a personal God, too. Human beings may grope toward God as if for a far-off subject, but in fact God "is not far from each one of us" (verse 27). God has chosen not to be remote and inaccessible, but readily available.

> *What does it mean to you to say that we live, move, and have our being in God? to think of God as "not far from each one of us"?*

REFLECT

The Inescapable God
Psalm 139
Who then are we? We are a people who cannot escape this God who wants to be in relationship with us and who will go to any and every length to be with us.

What's in the Bible?
Read Psalm 139. What phrases or ideas in this psalm speak most deeply to you? Why?

Psalm 139 expresses this intimate relationship that the Creator establishes with us. "You hem me in, behind and before, / and lay your hand upon me. . . . / It was you who formed my inward parts; you knit me together in my mother's womb (verses 5, 13). The person who wrote this psalm hints at a desire for escape from God (verse 7). The Bible presents us with people who find that they have walked into a story that was going on long before they arrived. They sometimes struggle with that, but in the end they find their authentic selves as they turn to God.

Prior to any choice that we make to follow God, there is a claim on our lives. It is built into us from before birth. We are "fearfully and wonderfully made" (verse 14), and we become the people we are meant to be when we are in relationship with the one who made us.

What are essential things about you that you didn't get to choose? How are those things gifts? If you could negotiate with God about these things, which would you give back and why?

Jesus at the Creation
John 1:1-5, 14

Maybe you have heard people talking about how they found their true selves when they found Jesus. The New Testament books of the Bible say things about Jesus that aren't said about any other human being. The Gospel of John begins the story of Jesus' life by going right back to the Creation.

What's in the Bible?
Read John 1:1-5, 14. What insights do you gain about human beings from this Bible reading? about God? about Jesus?

John 1 starts with the same words as Genesis: "In the beginning. . . ." John said that what was there at the beginning was the Word, a Greek way of talking about the ancient wisdom at the heart of the universe. Where the Bible differs from the Greeks, however, is in how it talks about the Word. The Word is Christ, God's chosen one, whom we know in Jesus. This Word is with God. The Word *is* God. The Word was in the words God spoke to create the universe; and now, with the coming of Jesus, the Word was in the world. "What has come into being in him was life," John said, "and the life was the light of all people" (verses 3-4).

> *What does the phrase "And the life was the light of all people" say to you about what it means to be a human being?*

REFLECT

It's just like God to do this. We see it in Genesis. There is God up to the elbows in connecting with man and woman. There is God like a potter working clay, making a person out of mud; like a craftsman working wood, building a woman from a rib. "And the Word became flesh and lived among us" (verse 14). Here is the astounding claim that God became human in Jesus and experienced the full range of human existence—loving, grieving, celebrating, weeping, suffering, and dying.

What does the phrase "And the word became flesh and lived among us" *say to you about God's regard for us?*

REFLECT

Finding Jesus and Finding Ourselves
Colossians 1:15-20
In the letter to the Colossians, Paul used language that is similar to the language in John in order to describe how we were created.

What's in the Bible?
Read Colossians 1:15-20. What phrases stand out for you in this Bible reading? Why? What does it say to you about the relationship between God and humans?

It is not simply that God made us and all the other creatures of the universe. It is not simply that there is purpose and intention in our creation. Paul went on to say that we were made *through Christ*. "All things have been created through him and for him. He himself is before all things, and in him all things hold together" (Colossians 1:16-17).

What this means for us is that if we are going to understand who we are, we can't just look inside. The essential fact about us is that God created us and we will only be able to understand what it means to be human in relationship with this God. Since everything hangs together in Christ, it is also true that we can't get a clear picture of ourselves without dealing with Christ. So there is more to self-discovery than listening to ourselves; we also have to listen for God.

All of this seems strange to our ears, especially if we have grown up in a culture that encourages us to define our identity apart from God. In US culture, we still celebrate the "self-made person": the immigrant who leaves behind the land he came from to start an entirely new life or the CEO who works her way to the top. Why should we bring God into this? Scientists can explain our existence without talking about the divine. People seem to be able to manage their lives quite easily without considering what it means to be God-created. There are plenty of people who do not understand why Jesus—this one particular historical figure from a backwater place in an ancient time—should make such a difference in determining their identity.

Augustine of Hippo, an early Christian leader and spiritual seeker, wrote this in the 5th century: "There is something of human beings that the very spirit of the individual that is within him or her does not know. But you, Lord, know all of each person, because you made us."[4] For Augustine this meant that even though we may have all that we need to be human, we cannot gain a full understanding of who we are until we seek out the God who made us.

A contemporary image for this might be a computer that comes loaded with the full version of a piece of software but that only lets you use part of it until you get a key code to unlock the rest of the program. You have the capacity to use the entire program only if you get in touch with the manufacturer. If you are like me, that does not mean you will then comprehend the whole program; but you will certainly have more access to it and will be able to have a richer experience of it. The people of the Bible affirm that we can best understand ourselves by seeking out our Maker who can lead us to a fuller experience of life.

> *What does it mean to you to hear that in Christ "all things hold together"? What connections do you make with this assertion and what it means to be a human being? How do you think we can discover who we are by listening to God? How do you listen to God? How do you respond to the image of a computer? What other images express the idea of getting in touch with our Maker?*

REFLECT

Something More

The Bible speaks to the part of us that knows that there is something more to our existence than what we can explain or do by our own efforts. All the scattered pieces of our lives demand a story to give them order. We sense that there is a reality more real than the one offered to us by our politics, our media, and even by our churches at times. Life is not flat; it is three-dimensional. The world is not a simple place to explain; it is full of complexity and wonder. The Bible invites us into a story that helps us glimpse what it means to be made by God.

Leif Enger, in his wonderful novel, *Peace Like a River,* creates a picture of a world only thinly separated from a larger, holy reality. Told from the perspective of an 8-year-old boy living in the northern plains of the United States, Enger's book is rich with images of a God-filled world breaking in for whoever has eyes to see it. There is pain and sorrow in his story, but it is always taking place within a landscape full of mystery and holiness. At one point he describes the stars in the sky as pinpoints of light shining through from another world.[5] The Bible is the root story for all stories like Enger's; it gives us a world where God is always present and always creating.

We might resist the Bible's story, though. We may accept that God has made the world but feel that our lives are so far from what they should be that it is hard to imagine that any of that image of God remains. *Maybe,* we wonder in our darker moments, *we are aliens who wander into this God-made world and don't have any claim on it. Maybe we do not deserve a share in this creation. Our lives are a mess. Surely God would have done better if we were really created the way the Bible says we were.*

The Bible refuses this interpretation. The hope in the Bible is in our God-connectedness. That is the point that it seeks to establish from the first chapter. There is trouble in paradise, and we see that in the Bible and in our lives; but it all happens with the words of God still echoing in the air: "This is good. This is very good."

In what ways do you sense something more in your life?

REFLECT

Here's Why I Care
How does the knowledge that you are God's good creation affect you? How will you listen for God this week? What will you do to try to develop a closer relationship with your Maker?

A Prayer
God of all creation, thank you for creating us. Thank you for reminding us who we are. Please continue to speak and create through our lives; in Christ, we pray. Amen.

---

[1] From *Lives to Offer: Accompanying Youth on Their Vocational Quest,* by Dori Grinenko Baker and Joyce Ann Mercer (The Pilgrim Press, 2007); page 71.
[2] Scripture taken from the Holy Bible, NEW INTERNATIONAL VERSION ®. Copyright © 1973, 1978, 1984 by International Bible Society. All rights reserved throughout the world. Used by permission of International Bible Society.
[3] From *God and the Rhetoric of Sexuality,* by Phyllis Trible (Augsberg Fortress Press, 1978).
[4] Adapted from *Confessions,* Books I-XIII, by Augustine, translated by F. J. Sheed (Hackett Publishing Company, 1993); page 176. For the purposes of this study, the writer of this publication has chosen to make the original quote inclusive. The original quote reads: "There is something of man that the very spirit of man that is in him does not-know. But you, Lord, know all of him, for you made him."
[5] From *Peace Like a River,* by Leif Enger (Grove Press, 2001); page 224.

Chapter Two

God Cares for Us

Bible Readings
Genesis 2:4–3:24; Hosea 11:1-11; Luke 12:22-31

The Questions
The Bible teaches us that God cares for us. Does God care for me? How can I trust that God cares? Does it matter? What difference does it make? Write responses to these questions in the space provided.

A Psalm

> Be mindful of your mercy, O Lord, and of your steadfast love,
>> for they have been from of old.
>
> Do not remember the sins of my youth or my transgressions;
>> according to your steadfast love, remember me,
>>> for your goodness' sake, O Lord! . . .
>
> All the paths of the Lord are steadfast love and faithfulness.
>
>> Psalm 25:6-7, 10

A Prayer

God of love and care, guide us as we explore more deeply what the Bible says about your care for us. Show us your love and your faithfulness and what it means in our lives; in Christ we pray. Amen.

Trust

The story of who we are as human beings has a lot to do with trust. We build our deepest relationships on trust, and our deepest wounds often come when that trust is broken. When we are able to trust that those around us care for us and that they have our best interests at heart, we thrive. When there is no trust and we experience pain from those near us, we start to doubt. What is real? Who am I? It is like travelling through a desert filled with mirages.

> *Who do you trust? When you have a secret or a story that you need to share, who do you tell? When you have a big decision to make, to whom do you turn?*

REFLECT

The Psalms are full of the raw emotions of people who lived on the edge of faith. If you read these songs you will see feelings of abandonment, despair, anger, and pain. Laced through them, however, is a continuing theme: God has not forgotten. God will redeem. God cares for us. Psalm 25:10 says, "All the paths of the Lord are steadfast love and faithfulness." *Chesed* is the Hebrew word that is translated "steadfast love" here; and it includes loyalty, unity, and deep connection. These are the things God promises throughout the Bible and the things we need most from God.

> *Read Psalm 25:6-10. Listen for what the person who wrote this psalm is asking of God. Imagine and write down what you think was happening in that life so many centuries ago that would lead to this prayer. Now spend a few minutes writing down what is happening in your life right now. How is your situation similar to the psalm writer? What is it that you want to ask of God?*

REFLECT

Hands-on Management
Genesis 2:4–3:24

If God created this world of wonders and got involved in it personally, how did it end up the way that it did? If God created us with so much potential and possibility, how did *we* end up the way we did?

What's in the Bible?
Read Genesis 2:4–3:24. What images or ideas stand out most for you in this Bible reading? What challenges you or makes you curious? What does the reading say to you about the man and the woman? about God? about God's care for the man and the woman?

Looking around at the world in the 18th century, great thinkers of the Enlightenment began to think that perhaps God had set up the store and then left it untended. The popular image was of the clockmaker who, with great skill and deftness, made a fine clock and then set it running, letting it tick on without any further involvement. If God is still around, they assumed, it is in a hands-off capacity.

By now you know that the Bible says something different about God. Looking through the opening chapters of Genesis, we saw a hands-on God who is intimately involved with the creatures that populate this new creation. Men and women are not just sent off to fend for themselves, even though they are given a great deal of freedom. As we saw, they have work to do. God charged them to cultivate the ground and to watch over it (Genesis 2:15). God gave them to each other and told them to flourish in their relationship together. God was present in the garden. The Bible talks about the Maker walking through the garden in the cool of the evening (3:8). Even though the world had been formed, time had begun, and work orders had been issued, God was going to stay around.

Things quickly got messy for the human beings, though. Even though they had been made in the image of God, they had a hard time living up to expectations. The only restriction that God placed on the man and the woman in the garden of Eden was that they should not eat from a particular tree, one with the tantalizing name: "the tree of the knowledge of good and evil" (2:16).

The storyteller of Genesis doesn't tell us why God put such a tree in the middle of the garden and then declared it off limits. We might wonder if God was leading them into temptation, like a parent setting a cookie jar in front of a child and saying, "There's something really good in this jar, but don't eat from it." However, everything we know about this God of the garden says that this divine being cares for what is created. God is all about goodness and flourishing. When God told Adam not to eat from the tree because he would die if he did so, we trust that this word, like all the other words the Creator has spoken, is a word of blessing.

> *How do you respond to God's instruction not to eat from the tree of the knowledge of good and evil? In what way could these words be a blessing?*
>
> **REFLECT**

This is the first hint in the Bible that there is darkness in the world. Amidst all the light and wonder of the dawning of time, there is also a shadow, something that we should pay attention to even if it comes under a desirable name such as *the knowledge of good and evil*. We could not call God a caring God if we did not listen to the blessings that come in the form of warnings.

You know this experience in your own life. As a young person growing up you heard the warnings of parents or other adults telling you that there is danger in the world. You likely experienced that at times as an unwelcome limitation or a series of no's: no drugs, no premarital sex, no smoking, no teasing your sister. However, usually a message of caring was behind the warnings and a desire that you not be hurt. When God says, "You will die if you eat from this tree," the rest of the story suggests that it is not a scare tactic to keep the man and woman down but a "care tactic" to keep them from the consequences of the world's darkness.

> *When have you experienced a scare tactic that turned out to be a "care tactic"?*

REFLECT

You know how we are, though. God must have foreseen what happened next, too, though this is the source of great debate in theological circles. Our knowledge of human nature tells us that it was probably inevitable that the tree with the tempting title was going to figure prominently in the story of humanity. In Genesis 3, we meet the tree.

We said earlier that Adam and Eve had a hard time living up to expectations, but perhaps a better way to explain the mess that results from this tree is to say that they were captivated by seemingly greater expectations. Because we have a capacity for wonder and a thirst for understanding who we are, we can wind up in some messy situations. The Bible doesn't explain the downfall of the first human beings by blaming something evil within us. The problems come because of the complexity of dealing with all the varied impulses coursing through us, a complexity we don't always handle well.

The conversation between the woman and the serpent is simple. In this enchanted time when snakes could talk, he used the gift of gab to put a seed of doubt in the mind of the woman by directly contradicting God. When she repeated God's command not to eat from the tree because they would die, the serpent said that it wasn't true. God was just afraid that the humans would become even greater than they already were. "You will not die; for God knows that when you eat of it your eyes will be opened, and you will be like God, knowing good and evil" (Genesis 3:4-5).

What happens next describes well the way in which we get ourselves into trouble by justifying our questionable actions. The Bible gives us a glimpse of what Eve was thinking, and what she thought about was how good the tree was. Like the other trees that God brought forth from the ground (2:9), this tree was good for food and it was a "delight to the eyes" (3:6). Moreover, the tree was desirable for something more than nourishment or beauty. Eve could see that it could make a person wise. So she ate the fruit from the tree. (It is often depicted as an apple, though the Bible doesn't say. I imagine a passion fruit.) Her husband, who was right there with her, ate too.

> *When have you rationalized a situation in order to justify a course of action? What happened?*
>
> REFLECT

Now God was presented with a problem. How would this caring God respond to creatures that had not trusted the words of warning and blessing? This new act showed that the humans had an unexpected capacity: They could use their God-given gifts to pursue something other than God. They could be deceived into believing that goodness, delight, and wisdom could be claimed apart from God. This is the moment to which the Bible points as the time when sin entered the world.

There it is. That word. *Sin.* You knew it had to be coming. Before we go any further, maybe you should spend a few minutes responding to that word because it has been used in so many different ways. Maye you've had it hurled at you by preachers, strangers, or friends. Maybe it stands like a huge hurdle to hearing anything else the Bible has to say about a caring God.

> *What do you think of when you hear the word* sin*?*
>
> REFLECT

Sin is a feature of human existence that occupies much of the rest of the Bible. It takes many forms in these pages. Sometimes the Bible describes sin as an external force plaguing humanity. Sometimes sin appears as the dark shadow lurking within us. It can show up as disobedience and brokenness and hurtfulness to oneself and others; but here at the beginning of the Bible we see its basic root. When human beings forget who they are and begin to give their lives to other stories about how the world works that do not reflect what God intends, then they begin to live apart from God. In the garden story of Genesis, we see that a deep separation had begun between the Lover of the Universe and the creatures called the Beloved. Would God still love them? Could God still love them?

The initial response seems harsh. God sent the man and woman out of the garden with warnings of pain and suffering to come. The woman would labor in childbirth, and the equality she experienced in her relationship with the man would now be tinged with the inequalities of power. The man would now have to struggle in his working of the land, and the original harmony he experienced with it as a creature of the earth was broken. Now he, and the woman with him, would experience death as they returned to the dust (3:16-19).

> *How do you respond to God's words and actions toward the man and the woman after their disobedience? What signs do you see of God's care in this part of the story?*

REFLECT

Even here, though, God's care remained. Though they were sent away from the garden, God replaced the fig leaf clothing they had put together to hide their nakedness with more substantial clothing made of animal skins; and the work they had been given to do continued. They were still sent forth "to till the ground" from which Adam was taken (3:23). The connection to the land would continue to be a source of blessing.

You probably know relationships between two people that seem to work despite factors that would doom other couples. Maybe one spouse is outgoing, extroverted, loud, and loves to go out dancing while the other is a much quieter homebody whose idea of a great night is staying home on the couch with an old movie and a bowl of popcorn. Perhaps the differences are more serious. One spouse or both has a volatile personality. One or both of them have had an affair. We politely say of such couples that they have a "complicated relationship." This is the picture the Bible gives us of the relationship between God and God's people. It is an understatement to say that it is complicated, but there are clear patterns. One of those patterns is the tendency of biblical characters to forget God's promises, to misunderstand their gifts and skills, to serve other gods who are not God, and to mistreat themselves and one another as a result.

> *What is your response to the use of the phrase* complicated relationship *to describe the relationship between God and humans?*
>
> REFLECT

In this way, the Bible is realistic. How many times have we found ourselves in situations where we recognize that we have forgotten we are God-created? How often have we been brought up short by the realization that we are limited? that the things the world values—what we look like, what we have, what we can buy—are ultimately empty? that we have hurt others and ourselves as a result? The pattern is established and familiar. Human beings are easily confused and often disconnected from God. Augustine of Hippo prayed, "Do Thou, O Lord my God, hear me and look upon me and see me and pity me and heal me, Thou in whose eyes I have become a question to myself and that is my infirmity."[1]

Loving the Child
Hosea 11:1-11

It's not just individuals who lose their way, though. The other consistent pattern that the Bible reveals about humans is that they are just as confused and disconnected in groups as they are on their own. Israel dominates the pages of the Scriptures as the chosen people of God, but they had a hard time living up to their identity. They quarreled with one another, they put their trust in other gods and other nations, and they had to be called back to their first love in God over and over.

What's in the Bible?
Read Hosea 11:1-11. What emotions do you identify in this Bible reading? What causes the emotions? What does the reading tell you about God's care for the people?

The result was a complicated relationship with God. The prophet Hosea was one of those who reminded the people of who they were and called them back. In Hosea 11, the prophet speaks for God and gives us an intimate picture of how God responded to the people's abandonment. It is as if God was a mother talking about her wayward son. "When Israel was a child, I loved him, / and out of Egypt I called my son," a reference to God's freeing the people from slavery some centuries before (verse 1).

Something had happened to the closeness of the relationship, though. The mother was calling Israel, but "the more I called them, the more they went from me" (verse 2). The sense of loss is clear as the mother recalled teaching Israel to walk, embracing the people in her arms, healing them, loving them, feeding them, and taking them up like an infant to her cheeks (verses 3-4). God grieved because God saw the result of the people's actions. Some would be taken back into Egypt. Others would be ruled by the reigning superpower of the time, Assyria. Violence would overtake them, and they would suffer.

> *If you are a parent, have you had such feelings toward your children? Do you remember such feelings from your parents or guardians? What does the image of the parent in this Bible reading say to you about God's care?*

REFLECT

In a way, this seems only right. After all, God had told them what the consequences of their actions would be. They were only getting what they deserved! However, here we find another clear pattern that tells us something about who God is: God is compassionate and wants to restore the people and redeem the relationship. Referring to the people now by names they would have known, God asked, "How can I give you up, Ephraim? How can I hand you over, Israel? / How can I make you like Admah? How can I treat you like Zeboiim?" (verse 8). In the end God said, "My compassion grows warm and tender. / I will not execute my fierce anger; I will not again destroy Ephraim; / for I am God and no mortal, the Holy One in your midst, and I will not come in wrath" (verses 8-9). Then God looked ahead to a day when "I will return them to their homes" (verse 11).

Where was the justice in that? How could God continue to stay connected to a people who refused to take care of themselves or to acknowledge the God who created and loved them? Why should God stick with us when we are so turned in on ourselves that we can't reach back to God? Well, it's a complicated relationship; but there is one simple thing about it: God remembers why we were created in the first place. God delights in us and cares for us. God knows what we are capable of. We can go astray, but we also have the capacity for love.

Bible Facts
Admah and Zeboiim were cities that were destroyed along with Sodom and Gomorrah (Deuteronomy 29:23).

> *Who in your life has modeled the love that is described in Hosea 11? What did they see in you that you perhaps weren't able to see in yourself? How have they reminded you of what you value and who you are? What did they do that helped you understand who you are and perhaps who God is? What would you like to tell them?*

The Problem of Trust
Luke 12:22-31

Even when we recognize that God is an incorrigible lover who just will not stop caring for us, we still have trouble responding to that love. One of our biggest hurdles is learning to trust that God will always be there and that the universe runs on God's love and not some other more uncaring or malicious force. The Bible gives us many portraits of people struggling to live with faith and trust in a caring God. They seem like people we know well. Usually they feel like us. As their stories reveal, the call of God is powerful but our own fears and worries get in the way. We think we have no one to rely on but ourselves, that our resources are limited, and that God has a limited sphere of influence.

> *What's in the Bible?*
> *Read Luke 12:22-31. How do you respond to Jesus' teaching in this parable? What images or ideas stand out for you? What challenges you? Why?*

Jesus confronted this struggle in his followers. He was preparing his disciples for a great adventure. Their lives were going to be turned around by their journey with Jesus. They were going out to tell others what God was doing, and they were going to face persecution for doing it. It was risky business, and the disciples were in denial about what they would have to give up.

The main thing they would have to let go of was their inability to trust. "Don't worry about your life," Jesus said, "what you will eat, or about your body, what you will wear" (Luke 12:22). Life is bigger than they could imagine. As long as they held on to these worries and made them the determining factors in their lives, they could never see that "life is more than food, and the body more than clothing" (verse 23). The ravens and the lilies have it right, and Jesus pointed them out as models. Birds and flowers grow in God's care, seemingly undisturbed about their ultimate end. We, on the other hand, miss the whole point of our existence when we confuse our daily needs with life itself.

It is easy to hold out on God. Trusting leaves us open to wounding, and many people have been hurt because they have placed their trust in others. Children who have been abused by adults they trusted, people betrayed by friends, lovers who have been abandoned, and even those who grieve the loss of a loved one can feel that their capacity to trust is damaged forever. How can we trust God, especially when those with a good sense of business would strongly disagree with Jesus' words?

Maybe it is because we sense that there is something more to us and to our lives than just food and clothing, than our sense of physical and material well-being. Some things have to be put at risk in order to live. Children grow up and leave home. We tell someone that we love him or her and open the closest held parts of ourselves for acceptance or rejection. People put their lives on the line for justice, for freedom, for their nation, and for their beliefs. Behind all of these is a trust that we will not find ourselves by holding ourselves back. We discover who we are by daring to trust that God cares and will bring us to a good end.

> *Worries are a constant part of our lives, and they can keep us attuned to what we need to be doing. However, Jesus seems to say that our worries can be a sign that we are holding ourselves back from God. Make a list of the things that you are worried about today. Which of these are realistic, and which are a sign of failing to trust God? How does the teaching of Jesus in Luke 12:22-31 communicate God's care for us?*

A Question of Reliability
Romans 8:31-39

How can we be assured that God is worthy of this trust? Where can we look to see evidence that God cares for us? The Christian Bible points to Jesus Christ as the best expression of who God is and what God intends for us.

> *What's in the Bible?*
> *Read Romans 8:31-39. How do you respond to Paul's words in this Bible reading? What does the reading say to you about God's care for us? about God's reliability?*

Paul, the early Christian missionary who influenced much of the way we think about and talk about Jesus, asked, "Who will separate us from the love of Christ? Will hardship, or distress, or persecution, or famine, or nakedness, or peril, or sword?" (Romans 8:35). These are important questions, because if we *can* be separated from God's love in Christ, then there are many things that are uncertain, including the question of how reliable God is.

Paul responded to his own questions, though, with a resounding no. It is clear where we stand with God. "Neither death, nor life, nor angels, nor rulers, nor things present, nor things to come, nor powers, nor height, nor depth, nor anything else in all creation, will be able to separate us from the love of God in Christ Jesus our Lord" (verses 38-39). Paul was convinced of this because God came in Jesus, and the story of Jesus' life is one in which he faced all the challenges Paul laid out, from hardship to nakedness to sword, and even in death showed how God's love is victorious. A God who goes that far to share in our lives and to experience our infirmities is not a God who takes our rejection as the final word. God continues to reach out and claim the world and the people that have been God's beloved from the beginning of all things.

What do you believe is separating you from the love of God?
What are your obstacles to trusting God? other people?

Yes, God Cares

Nobody ever said that fate cared about us. If we live in a world without God, there is no reason we should expect that there is a rhyme or a reason to the trajectory of our lives. However, if the Bible is right, then we are connected at a deep level to a passionate God who does care about us. What do you do with a God like that?

> *What difference does it make if the world is infused with God's love? Who are you if one of the things you have to say about yourself is that God loves you?*
>
> **REFLECT**

> *Here's Why I Care*
> *What learning or insights in the Bible readings and content of this chapter have meant most to you? Why? Write endings to the following sentences: Because God loves the world, I am going to ____. Because God loves me, I am going to ____.*
>
> **HERE'S WHY I CARE**

A Prayer

God, we give you thanks for your care, for your steadfast love no matter what. Teach us to accept your love and to express it in our lives; in Christ we pray. Amen.

---

[1] From *Confessions;* page 198.

Chapter Three

God Saves Us

Bible Readings
Exodus 1–4; Luke 2:25-38; 19:1-10; Romans 6:3-12; Ephesians 1:5-12; Colossians 3:1-4; Hebrews 2:6-12

The Questions
What does it mean to say that God saves us? Do we need to be saved? From what? How does the word *salvation* apply to contemporary life?

A Psalm

> The Lord is my rock, my fortress, and my deliverer,
>> my God, my rock in whom I take refuge,
>> my shield, and the horn of my salvation, my stronghold.
> I call upon the Lord, who is worthy to be praised,
>> so I shall be saved from my enemies.
>>> Psalm 18:2-3

A Prayer

The Bible says you save your people, God, but there are so many things that stand between the world and salvation. There are many bogs and mighty waters. Show us what salvation means; in Christ we pray. Amen.

Confidence and Disability

Who are all these confident people that stride through life as if they haven't a care in the world? These people on our television screens, leading seminars, giving us professional advice—are they as confident as they seem? Because you and I know that there are all sorts of reasons for us (and them!) to feel insecure. We often feel like we are mired in mud or overwhelmed by stormy seas. We are looking for a deliverer.

What does your miry bog or troubled water look like today? Where are you feeling the need for a savior? Take a minute to draw the scene (or to draw what it feels like) or to describe it in a few words.

REFLECT

What would you give to be desirable? Would you consider an extreme makeover? plastic surgery? an image consultant? Would you hire an agent? Would you puff your résumé? doctor your photo for an online dating service? All of these options suggest that we can't handle the truth—or at least we're afraid that others can't handle the truth about us. There are just too many things we would like to conceal: the physical features we would gladly trade away, the bad habits we've fallen into, the self-doubt that gnaws at our self-confidence, the things we've done that we would like to undo, the resolutions we've made to do better that are still waiting for our resolve.

One of the most surprising things about the Bible is that it makes almost no effort to cover over the flaws in the people it describes. Even the greatest kings and most powerful prophets appear with their slips showing. King David, the most celebrated of all of Israel's rulers, had an adulterous affair and ordered the death of an innocent man as a result (1 Samuel 11–12). Jonah, called by God to preach to the city of Ninevah, turned out to be fearful, rebellious, and petulant He ran in the other direction and ended in the belly of a big fish! Paul, the great apostle of the Christian era, was an approving bystander of murderous mobs before his conversion; and even after he started following Jesus, he admitted to doing things that he did not want to do because the effects of sin were still there working on him and in him (Romans 7:14-25).

One of the even more surprising things about the Bible, though, is that it tells us that despite the way these people acted, they were still desirable to God. God did not give up on them no matter how bad they acted, no matter how desperate they were, and no matter how hopeless they seemed. It is as if God is determined to save us despite ourselves.

> *In what areas would you like to be more confident or desirable? What would you change about yourself? Why?*
>
> **REFLECT**

Who Are My People?
Exodus 1–2

Moses is one of those human characters we meet in the Bible. He was born into a Hebrew slave family in Egypt at a time of great threat.

What's in the Bible?
Read Exodus 1–2. Which characters stand out most for you? Why? How do you respond to Moses? How is he portrayed in the Bible reading? What connections do you make between this Bible reading and the idea of salvation or being saved?

Pharaoh, ruler of the land, had ordered that all male infants of the Hebrews should be drowned in the river Nile; but Moses was a child of promise. He was saved from death by the intervention of a compassionate mother, a faithful sister, and Pharaoh's own daughter, who adopted him into the royal family when she found him floating in the river in the basket his mother had prepared for him.

The boy grew up with an uncertain identity. He was never fully part of the Egyptian people who had claimed him, and yet he was also not one of the Hebrews. It became painfully clear how torn he was one day when, as a young man, he went out among "his people," the Hebrews, who were laboring under the Egyptian overlords. Moses' sense of justice was inflamed when he saw an Egyptian beating "one of his kinsfolk." Moses responded by striking the slave master and killing him. Not being good at the art of hiding his mistakes, he buried the body in the sand. When the murder was found out and the Hebrews, "his own people," questioned his actions, he fled for the distant land of Midian, where he thought his days in Egypt were done.

> **Bible Facts**
> The name *Moses* is part of a compound in Egyptian names as a root meaning "son of." In the early part of his life, this was an open question for Moses. Would he be a child of the Egyptians or the Hebrews? When he arrived in Midian fleeing from what he had done, he was called an Egyptian. It took an encounter with God on a mountain to settle the question that the God of the Hebrews was going to give Moses his identity, too.[1]

Accept That You Are Accepted
Exodus 3:1–4:20

A great theologian of the 20th century, Paul Tillich, once entitled a sermon "You Are Accepted." The sentence could be addressed to Moses. Moses might have thought he was done with Egypt, but God was not done with Moses. After he had married and settled into life as a desert shepherd, God found him on a mountaintop and called him to return to the scene of the crime.

> *What's in the Bible?*
> *Read Exodus 3:1–4:20. What images, words, or phrases stand out for you in this Bible reading? What does the reading say to you about Moses' personality? about God? about God's relationship with Moses? with the Hebrews?*

The famous story of God speaking to Moses from a burning bush shows the persistence with which God reaches out to people who thought their journeys were through or already predetermined. Moses' body language said it all. He hid his face because he was afraid to look at God. "Surely," he must have thought to himself, "a person who has done the unholy things that I have done cannot survive the presence of a holy God."

This was not the end of Moses, though. In many ways, it was only the beginning. God had work for him to do in leading the people out of slavery. Moses, for his part, had a number of objections. The first was revealing. "Who am I that I should go to Pharaoh and lead the people out of Egypt?" (Exodus 3:11). There were other objections. He wanted to know God's name, wanted some evidence of God's authority to take with him, and he claimed he could not speak well. (Given his performance here I doubt that claim!) However, it seems that the biggest problem Moses had was in believing that God wanted to use him.

> *What are you not doing that you would be doing if you believed that God wanted to use you? What keeps you from hearing that God has a greater purpose for you?*

God wasn't just seeking out Moses, though. Moses' salvation was tied up in what God wanted for his whole people. The Bible says that God heard the groaning of the people in slavery and remembered the relationship established with their ancestors. God had looked upon the people and taken notice of them (Exodus 2:23-25). They were still the people after God's own heart. They were still the object of God's desire, so God set out to save them.

"I have observed the misery of my people who are in Egypt," God told Moses. "I have heard their cry on account of their taskmasters. Indeed, I know their sufferings, and I have come down to deliver them from the Egyptians, and to bring them up out of that land to a good and broad land, a land flowing with milk and honey" (3:7-8). The rest of the Exodus story shows the extent to which God would go to bring the people out. It is a dramatic and troubling story. Rivers would be fouled with blood, seas would part, armies would be routed, and death would come to the Egyptian households; but the Hebrews would be saved.

It is a story that is repeated throughout the Hebrew Scriptures. There are high moments when the relationship between God and the people seemed secure, when the people were faithful to the promise God held out for them and they were a blessing to the nations. There were many more moments, however, when the people forgot their connection to God and lost their way. They turned to other gods. They neglected the plight of the poor, the vulnerable, and the immigrants in their midst. They were defeated by other kingdoms and carried off into exile. Each time God turned to them and reminded them who they were. God saved them by remembering a name. When Moses asked, "Who shall I say has sent me?" God gave an enigmatic name, "I AM WHO I AM." Then God said, "Thus you shall say to the Israelites, 'The LORD, the God of your ancestors, the God of Abraham, the God of Isaac has sent me to you'" (3:14-15). The word LORD is used for the Hebrew that is the divine name, a form of the verb *to be*. It means something like the One "who is" and "who will be." How God acts in the Bible reveals who God is. The God who saves us is the God who acts in our midst, who knows our names, and who identifies with us.

Who are the forgotten people in your community who need the God who will take up their name and their cause? How are you being called to identify yourself with them?

REFLECT

Salvation in a Child's Form
Luke 2:25-38

Perhaps you can imagine one of those downtrodden Hebrew slaves awaiting a savior. It's a familiar position for people whose lives have become defined by defeat and depression. Where do you look when the ruling powers of the day refuse to release you? Does your soul dry up, or do you find ways to sustain hope?

What's in the Bible?
Read Luke 2:25-38. What images, words, or ideas in the Bible reading particularly stand out for you? Why? What is your impression of Simeon? of Anna? How do you respond to their view of God's saving power through the infant Jesus?

In the Gospel of Luke we have the story of two elderly prophets who met the infant Jesus as he was brought into the Temple to be dedicated to God. Simeon was the first to see the child. A faithful Jew, he had been waiting for the Messiah, the one anointed by God to save the people. The Bible says that the Holy Spirit, which had guided the prophets in older times, had come on Simeon as well and had assured him that he would live to see the promised Savior. When he saw Jesus' parents bringing the Infant into the Temple, he went to them, took the Child in his arms, and said, "Master, now you are dismissing your servant in peace, according to your word; / for my eyes have seen your salvation" (Luke 2:29-30). To see the Child was enough. Simeon could see the promise of a new day—and not just for his people but for the whole world. To see Jesus was enough to know that the end of the story was going to be assured.

Anna was the other prophet, a woman who had been widowed at a young age and who had dedicated her life to worship at the Temple. She joined Simeon and began to preach, interpreting for all those around what Jesus' coming meant. In Jesus they saw that God remained faithful to Israel, that God identified with the suffering of the world, and that God entered the world to save.

What does the story of Simeon and Anna say to you about God's relationship with us?

REFLECT

A Taxman Finds Jesus
Luke 19:1-10

Though it happened in fits and starts, people were seeing the promise of salvation in Jesus throughout his journeys. Fishermen dropped nets to follow him. Women broke social conventions of the day to talk with him and wash his feet. Those in need of sight and those with shattered lives and bodies found healing in his presence. Mostly people discovered who they were in God's eyes through Jesus' challenge to them and acceptance of them.

What's in the Bible?

Read Luke 19:1-10. What stands out for you in this story? What does it say to you about God's relationship to people?

No one had a more dramatic experience of salvation than Zacchaeus, a small man who served as one of the hated tax collectors in the city of Jericho. People assumed that tax collectors were corrupt representatives of the state who would abuse their position for personal gain. As a rich man, Zacchaeus certainly seemed to have taken advantage of the opportunities.

When Jesus came through town, however, Zacchaeus was not squireled away plotting how to add to his ill-gotten gains. Instead he was up a tree trying to get a glimpse of who this Jesus was that was causing such a stir on his way to Jerusalem. Imagine his consternation when Jesus stopped beneath his tree, looked up at the man perched unsteadily on a limb, and said, "Zacchaeus, hurry and come down; for I must stay at your house today" (Luke 19:5).

It didn't make the crowd happy. They grumbled about Jesus' choice of dinner companions. "He has gone to be a guest of one who is a sinner" (verse 7). However, Jesus' willingness to receive and to be received by one of the most suspect members of the community seems to have had a big impact on Zacchaeus. He pledged on the spot to give half of his possessions to the poor and to make restitution four times over to any one he had defrauded. That's when Jesus surprised everyone by saying that on that day salvation had come to Zacchaeus's house because "he too is a son of Abraham" (verse 9). Zacchaeus's actions revealed that he had been transformed by encountering Jesus. He had found his identity in the story of God's people going all the way back to God's covenant with Abraham (Genesis 12:1-3). Zacchaeus the despised tax collector was God's child.

What changes would you make in your life if you accepted that you were a child of God and loved without reservation?

REFLECT

The Significance of the Tree
Hebrews 2:6-13

A sycamore tree plays an important role in the story of Zacchaeus's salvation. Another kind of tree is important to how Christians tell the story of salvation: the cross.

> ### What's in the Bible?
> *Read Hebrews 2:6-13. How do you respond to this Bible reading? What feelings or thoughts do you have about it? What challenges you or makes you curious? What words or phrases stand out for you? Why?*

In the story the Bible tells, Jesus' death on the cross is the defining moment of God's saving work. All four Gospels culminate with this act in which Jesus is betrayed by friends, handed over to the authorities of the day, beaten and humiliated, and then nailed to a cross—an execution method favored by the Romans. Yes, it is a gruesome story; and it has caused many people through time to wonder why such a bloody means was necessary for salvation.

Why should Jesus be any different from any of us? Not all of our deaths are as dramatic or as tortured as his, but they are unavoidable. If God were going to come into the world and share in our every human experience, then death of some kind would be inevitable. The drama of his death is a result of a human tendency to misunderstand love.

Hebrews 2:6-13 describes how Jesus came to live out what it means to be a true human being. When we want to know what it means for us to be human, made "for a little while lower than angels" [Hebrews 2:7]), we can look to Jesus. It is only right that his life should be one that looks like ours and therefore only "fitting" that he should become the pioneer in salvation by enduring suffering and death.

However, Jesus is more than a model for us. Because he is God and human he shows us that we are not only sufferers, we are also children—and more than children, brothers and sisters with Jesus (verses 10-13); and because Jesus is who he is, the sin that nailed him to the cross was shown ultimately to have no power over those who are God's children.

What do you feel when you look at the cross? How do you understand the meaning of the suffering that Jesus endured? What difference does it make to think of Jesus' death as opening up a way for you into the life of God?

Alive to God in Jesus Christ
Romans 6:3-11

The later books of the New Testament devote a lot of space to praising the risen Jesus. If the cross reminds us of how God entered the suffering of the world and did not ignore the awful things that can happen in us and to us because of sin, the empty tomb that signaled Jesus' resurrection from the dead tells us why Christians have hope. Paul, the writer of the Letter to the Romans, knows that we find our true worth in the love that raised Jesus from the dead.

What's in the Bible?
Read Romans 6:3-11. What images, words, or phrases stand out for you in the Bible reading? What challenges you or makes you curious? Why?

The Gospel stories tell us that when Jesus was baptized in the Jordan River the skies split, a dove descended, and a voice from heaven said, "You are my Son, the Beloved; with you I am well pleased" (Mark 1:11). The love that enfolded Jesus was so great that it overflows into the love of God for all humanity.

That ordinary-looking water with which Christians are sprinkled or in which they are dunked at baptism becomes an entry into a great mystery. They are "baptized into Christ Jesus." They go under the water as a way of dying with Christ and emerge from the water as a way of sharing in the new life Christ has wrested from death. They then become people forever identified with Jesus. You are no longer a person defined by the worst you have done but a person defined by what God knows you can be. "You also must consider yourselves dead to sin and alive to God in Christ Jesus," Paul said (Romans 6). We are not condemned. Where is the good news in that identity? We are saved, and therefore we can begin to live like it.

What is the obstacle that keeps you from claiming your identity as God's child? that keeps you from experiencing what it means to be "alive to God in Christ Jesus"?

There's No Place Like Home
Ephesians 1:3-12

In the Letter to the Ephesians, Paul says that we are blessed and God intends for us a holy and blameless relationship of love through Christ.

What's in the Bible?
Read Ephesians 1:3-12. What words, phrases, or images speak to you in this Bible reading? Why? How do you respond to the idea of adoption? What connections do you see between adoption and salvation?

The Letter to the Ephesians uses the language of adoption to describe the way God saves us and makes us part of the family of God. It is as if we have been lost and disconnected and are looking for home. Through the love shown on the cross and God's willingness to give life itself for us, we are given a place and an inheritance.

The longing for a home is a deep one in us. Even those of us who grow up in loving families often have the feeling that we are searching for another place of acceptance and nurture. We wander through strange lands, like Dorothy Gale in *The Wizard of Oz,* wondering how we will find home and who will help us reach it. We want to trust that there is a love at the center of the universe large enough to include us. We want to believe that all the broken pieces of our lives will somehow be taken up and remade, like some great mosaic mural, into something beautiful.

In the Ephesians passage we see the beauty beyond the suffering. In Christ, God gathers up all the broken things of earth and heaven and reveals a divine intention. Our home is in Christ. We won't be left alone to our own devices. We won't be enslaved to our sin or the sin of the world.

> *When have you felt the need to go home? What was it like? How do you connect this idea with salvation?*

Putting on New Clothes and Christ
Colossians 3:1-14

It was not until I entered college that I bought my first clothes on my own. Being fairly oblivious to fashion as a teen, I was quite content to let my mother be my image consultant and buyer. Then came the day when I went looking for some shirts at a time when I was having deep relationship problems that made me doubt myself and my desirability. I emerged from the store with two shirts that were the height of '80's style. They had no sleeves, and I felt they showed off my muscles. To me they said, "I am strong, confident, and tough." I was pleased at how I felt when I put on one of these shirts. This was not "retail therapy." My issues were not resolved because I had a new piece of clothing, but believing that I was perceived differently began to change my self-perception. I was on the way to claiming something that I had already but had not been able to claim. It was a step toward integrity and strength.

What's in the Bible?
Read Colossians 3:1-14. What words, phrases, and images stand out for you in this reading? How do you respond to the image of clothing?

Paul uses the image of putting on new clothes to describe what it means to live out our salvation as children of God who are created in the image of God (Colossians 3:10). The Letter to the Colossians tells us that God knows who we are. It uses past tense verbs to describe the state of the Christian. We "have died" and "have been raised with Christ"; and because of that, the things that once bound us no longer have power. God knows better than we do what we are capable of. We can be blind to our potential because of our fears and our wounds and our misguided estimations of ourselves; but God sees what to us is hidden, and Colossians says that "your life is hidden with Christ in God" (verse 3). When Christ is revealed to us at the end of all things, then we also will be revealed like some great masterpiece of art waiting to be unveiled. The promise to you is that you are going to look good on that day with a beauty that belongs to Christ.

What connections do you make between the idea that God saves us and the idea of clothing ourselves with new behaviors? What new clothes of a life in Christ would you like to wear?

God's Vision of Us

So perhaps beside the mirrors we look in each morning we should place a picture of Jesus, knowing that the beauty we see in him is the same beauty that God can see in us. Maybe you resist that idea because you do not believe you are worthy to be seen that way. *Who am I to be saved by God?* you might wonder. However, the Bible suggests a different question, "Who are you *not* to be saved by God?"

God has funny tastes. The Bible is full of stories of how God takes unexpected people such as Moses, Esther, and Paul and turns them into reluctant heroes. Somehow desirability is in the eye of the beholder; and once these people accepted that God had chosen them despite themselves to walk into a new day, they began to live like the men and women God knew they could be. So can we.

Here's Why I Care

What keeps you from seeing yourself as the apple of God's eye? How can the knowledge that God saves us make a difference to you? How can you live clothed in God's care and salvation in the week ahead?

A Prayer
Saving God, we give you thanks that you save us, day by day, through Jesus Christ. Help us live in the love and hope of your saving ways; in Christ we pray. Amen.

---

[1] From *The Storyteller's Companion to the Bible,* Vol. 2, Exodus-Joshua, Michael E. Williams, editor (Abingdon Press, 1992); page 30.

Chapter Four

God Invites Us Into Relationship

Bible Readings
Genesis 15; Joshua 24:1-27; Matthew 19:16-22; Acts 2:41-47; 1 Corinthians 1:3-9; 2 Corinthians 5:18-21; 1 John 1:1-7

The Questions
The Bible reveals that we are invited into relationship with God. What does that mean? How do we have a relationship with God? What difference will it make in our lives?

A Psalm

Protect me, O God, for in you I take refuge.

I say to the Lord, "You are my Lord;

    I have no good apart from you.

        Psalm 16:1-2

A Prayer

God, be with us and guide us as we explore the meaning and value of your invitation into relationship with you. Help us to hear your invitation, and show us how we can respond; in Christ we pray. Amen.

The Desire for Relationship

Do you remember your first crush? Maybe you remember daydreaming in class writing the name of that special someone all over your notebook. In a different generation you might have carved your name in a tree along with your beloved's, the obligatory plus sign between the names telling the story. You didn't care who knew; what was important was that you cared to be known as the person who loves Dawn or Eddie or Maria.

A consistent hunger of the human heart is the desire for deep relationship. It is so engrained in us that we often introduce ourselves to others based on our personal connections. In small, rural places it is still common to have people do their introductions based on family trees. "Oh, you know Leon. He's Hattie's grandson."

Maybe that is why the Bible spends so much time talking about relationships as well. To talk about who we are in biblical terms is to talk about the people to whom we are related. Primarily it is to talk about how our whole existence and identity is tied up in God.

What relationships in your life mean most to you? Why? How do they help you understand who you are? How is God with you in these relationships?

God Initiates Covenant
Genesis 15

Ionthe Rhodes is something of a legend where I live. At an age when many are beginning to think about their retirement, she did something that no other person had ever done before. She put on her swimsuit, jumped in the water, and swam the mouth of the Chesapeake Bay. The 15-mile crossing is the Virginia equivalent of swimming the English Channel. Who knows what called her to do such a thing at her age, but something told her that her journey wasn't over. There was a new adventure waiting for her in that wide expanse of water. Rhodes went on to teach many more youth and adults how to swim after that day and worked tirelessly for the American Red Cross.[1]

When have you taken on a challenge or an adventure that seemed unexpected to those who knew you or even to yourself? What did you learn about yourself or about God through the experience?

One consistent message that comes through in the Bible is that God is continually inviting people into new journeys and new relationships that they could not have foreseen before God came along. Even people who thought their stories were nearly done are suddenly launched in surprising directions by this God who does not know how to leave well enough alone. Take Abram and Sarai. At a rather advanced age (Abram was 75, Sarai only ten years younger), God called them to continue a journey that Abram's father had begun. "Leave your country, your people and your father's household and go to the land I will show you," God said to Abram (Genesis 12:1, NIV). God promised the childless couple descendants and told them that they would be a blessing to the nations. There were obvious questions to be asked here such as how this would happen; but initially Abram responded like Ionthe Rhodes, jumping off into the unknown with all that he had.

What's in the Bible?
Read Genesis 15. What stands out for you in this Bible reading? What challenges you or makes you curious? Why? What does it say to you about God? about Abram? about the relationship between them?

Later, when Abram and Sarai had become established in this promised land and had some history with God, Abram received the promise again. "Do not be afraid, Abram," the Lord said. "I am your shield; your reward shall be very great" (15:1). Abram knew that there were huge problems with this divine blessing. For one thing, God had promised children and offspring; but Sarai's biological clock had long since stopped ticking. Abram was not a great candidate for fatherhood himself. God's response was to take Abram out beneath the night sky carpeted with stars. "Look toward heaven and count the stars, if you are able to count them . . . so shall your descendants be" (verse 5).

Not only did Abram question the promise of offspring, he questioned the possession of the land (verse 8). How could he be assured that God would uphold the promise? His was just one family in a region of competing kings and armies.

God responded with a covenant, a binding agreement to accompany Abram and his children on a long and difficult trail that would eventually lead back to this land. The covenant ceremony was gory. A heifer, a goat, a ram, and two birds were slaughtered with all but the birds cut in half and placed on either side of a makeshift pathway. As the sun set, Abram fell into a heavy sleep and a fearful darkness descended on the scene. It was the kind of sleep that overcame Adam as God took a rib and created a woman (2:21). Once again God was going to initiate a new kind of relationship for humanity.

As Abram slept, God spoke into the deep knowing of his dreams and described the journey that was to come in which Abram's descendants would move to slavery in a foreign land and then to deliverance and return. Then in the growing darkness, a light appeared as a smoking pot and a flaming torch began to move down the path between the animal parts. It was God putting a seal on the promise. Abram could be assured of God's presence because they were now in a life and death relationship that God would not abandon. God made a unilateral covenant with Abram and his descendants. Regardless of the faithfulness or failure of the human partners, God would maintain the covenant.

What does the covenant God initiated with Abram say to you about the relationship between God and human beings?

Bible Facts
The covenant ceremony described in Genesis 15 was typical of the way solemn agreements were formalized in the ancient Near Eastern culture. People making covenants with one another would walk through the halves of slaughtered animals and vow to uphold their end of the bargain. The sacrificed animals were reminders of how seriously they took the vow. In effect they were saying, "May I end up like these creatures if I don't keep my word."[2]

"Gotta Serve Somebody"
Joshua 24:1-27

We have already seen how the Bible portrays a God who seeks out and saves human beings. From the earliest stories of Genesis we can see how God desires a partnership with human beings. Abram and Sarai's experience with God shows how that partnership was deepened through covenant. God took on the identity of a particular family and asked them to walk alongside this surprising deity. You have to admit it is an unusual move. The Creator of the universe decided to be known as the God of Abraham (the name by which Abram was eventually known). Why would God decide to take *our* name?

Of course, the relationship was meant to be mutual. Though God made the first move in establishing the covenant, the Bible tells us about many other times when the people were invited to bind themselves to God. Joshua issued one of the strongest challenges to covenant with God.

What's in the Bible?
Read Joshua 24:1-27. What particularly strikes you about this Bible reading? What makes you curious? How do you respond to Joshua's retelling of God's actions on behalf of God's people as the basis for choosing to serve God?

Having taken up the mantle of leadership from Moses, Joshua had led the former Hebrew slaves into the land promised to Abraham once again. Centuries had passed since that dark night of God's covenant with Abraham. All of the things that God had promised had come to pass. With the people now occupying the land, Joshua told them that they faced a choice. They could claim and serve this God who had claimed them or they could serve the other gods of the land. "As for me and my household," Joshua said, "We will serve the LORD" (Joshua 24:15).

The world of the Bible doesn't leave much room for middle ground in serving God. In our contemporary world many say that it is possible to live without a relationship to a divine being. People can and do say, "I don't serve any god." This is a suspect statement from a biblical perspective. We may not serve the God of Israel, but there are all sorts of things that claim our reverence and service. As human beings we have an innate need to give ourselves to something beyond ourselves, so we place our lives at the service of our nation, our true love, our addiction, or our favorite sports team among many other things.

Joshua confronts us with an ultimate choice. He sounds a bit like Bob Dylan singing "Gotta Serve Somebody." We are created to be related; and we can live that out in ways that bring us closer to God, or we can live it out in ways that do damage to others and ourselves.

Create a chart that tracks the way you have spent your time in the past week. You are not trying to picture a typical week or an ideal week, just the actual week gone by. In what activities did you participate, and how long did you spend at each? Include time spent sleeping and eating. Imagine someone else looking at this chart. To what or whom would they say you were giving your life? If you wanted to choose with Joshua and his household to serve God, what would change about this chart (and your life)?

No Holding Back
Matthew 19:16-22

Jesus is as demanding as Joshua. The choices he presents to people are stark. He met a group of fishermen working their nets on a lake and told them to drop everything and follow him (Luke 5:1-11). He saw a tax collector named Matthew and told him to leave his tables (Matthew 9:9). He looked out to a crowd of would-be disciples and said, "If any want to become my followers, let them deny themselves and take up their cross and follow me. For those who want to save their life will lose it, and those who lose their life, for my sake, and for the sake of the gospel, will save it" (Mark 8:34-35). There is no holding back. To find their lives, Jesus' followers have to give up what they know of themselves to receive their true selves.

What's in the Bible?

Read Matthew 19:16-22. What stands out for you in the Bible reading? What does it tell you about the young man? about Jesus?

The challenge is clear in the story of Jesus and a wealthy young man. The man had come to see what it would take for him to win eternal life. Initially, Jesus told him to keep the commandments. The man persisted. "Which ones?" When Jesus replied with several of the Ten Commandments and with the teaching about loving neighbor as oneself, the man objected. "I have kept all these; what do I still lack?" He had followed the rules. He had obeyed the commandments set out in the law of Moses. What more did he need to do?

Jesus saw right to the heart of what he was holding back. "Sell your possessions, and give the money to the poor," he said, "then come, follow me" (Matthew 19:21). For the young man it was too much. Unlike the fishermen and Matthew, he could not drop the things that had given his life meaning and identity before Jesus came along. He turned away with a heavy heart and did not follow Jesus.

What might you have to leave behind if Jesus were to come calling? Imagine Jesus finding you with one of those dear attachments that keep you from being who you are supposed to be. What does the scene look like? Write about or draw it.

REFLECT

Invitation Into Community Relationship
Acts 2:38-47

The story of the rich young man tells us something else about how Jesus transforms our identity. Not only do we understand our relationship to God through Jesus' call, but we also have a new relationship with other people. We are part of a new community of people who are connected to one another and who have a new way of relating to the world. When the young man turned around to go home, he was not only retreating behind the barrier his possessions posed, but he was also missing the opportunity to be part of a new fellowship. Jesus' followers constituted a new way of being in the world.

What's in the Bible?
Read Acts 2:38-47. What images or ideas stand out for you in this Bible reading? What challenges you? Why? How do you respond to the communal life of these early believers?

In Acts 2:38-47, Peter, on behalf of Christ, invites the people to repent and be baptized into a new community empowered by the Holy Spirit. The church they formed would have been considered radical in any age. They were so intimately connected with one another that they began to practice communal living with individuals selling their private property and putting what they had at the service of the larger community. When they accepted God's invitation for relationship through Jesus Christ, they not only entered into the life of Jesus Christ, but they were also initiated into a new relationship with brothers and sisters they didn't even know they had. They began to pray together, eat together, and to serve one another. They were no longer strangers but family.

When I imagine what this community must have been like, I remember a small home in Cortazár, a small city in the high deserts of central Mexico. I was there in the fall of 2001, shortly after the September attacks on the World Trade Center and the Pentagon. A small group of us were meeting with pastors and churches throughout the area, planning for work teams that would come in the next year. The Balderas family had been kind enough to open their home to me.

It was an emotional week. At a church service I had been surrounded by members of the Mexican congregation who prayed for me and the other *norteamericanos* and for the grief we were experiencing as a result of the attacks. I had not even known how much I needed to grieve until these fellow Christians helped me see it. I cried for the first time since 9/11.

Later, I was sitting in the front room of the Balderas house, which during the day was open as a fruit stand. I sat among the avocados and tomatillos helping one of the children with her English homework. The rest of the family was gathered with us around a television with fading signal watching the seventh game of the World Series. Though my Spanish was weak, I suddenly had a powerful experience of belonging. Only a church formed by Jesus Christ had brought about this unlikely communion. Since then I have believed that, whatever the new community Jesus initiates looks like, it smells of lime and cilantro. And there is baseball.

What does family smell like for you? When has a gathering of people who were not a community before become an experience of belonging for you? What made that experience important? Write down memories from that occasion or draw it.

The Fellowship Of Jesus
1 Corinthians 1:3-9

You might be saying, "What happened? Where is the church of Acts?" It is true that for every story of Christians sharing their resources and helping those in need, for every time of connection in a fragrant Mexican fruit stand, there are many other stories of Christians not "getting it" and failing to live out their baptisms. In fact, the problems were on display early on. When Paul wrote to the communities of Christians he had helped establish, he was often writing to address conflicts and misunderstandings that had grown up among the new followers of Jesus. His surviving letters that have been collected in the New Testament still resonate with us because we know how fragile human community is.

What's in the Bible?
Read 1 Corinthians 1:3-9. What stands out for you in this Bible reading? What does it say to you about Paul? about God? about the invitation to relationship with God through Jesus Christ?

The Christians in the city of Corinth were a particularly conflicted group. Paul's first and second letters to the Corinthians reveal a community that could fight over just about anything: spiritual pride, sexual behavior, competing leaders, and how to relate to the rest of the world, among other things. Paul spoke directly to these problems, but he framed them within a message of confidence.

In the introduction to the first letter, Paul told the community, "God is faithful; by him you were called into the fellowship of his Son, Jesus Christ our Lord" (1 Corinthians 1:9). In other words, God had invited them into relationship with God through Jesus Christ. God's grace had been given to them in Christ Jesus. They did not lack for any gift that they might have needed to be the people God called them to be. Divided as they were (something that becomes clear as early as verse 11 of the first chapter!), they were part of a fellowship—not just the fellowship of Corinth but the fellowship of Jesus, in whom they found their identity.

Christians are sometimes chided for their tendency to emphasize their relationship to Jesus as if nothing else were happening. The Christian message has, at times, been reduced to "Me and Jesus have our own thing going." However, like spokes going toward the center of a wagon wheel, the closer we get to Jesus, the closer we find ourselves to other people seeking the same center. When we respond to the invitation to relationship with God through Jesus, we find that Jesus is more than an individual; he is a fellowship (verse 9).

> *What images or thoughts come to mind when you hear the words* relationship with Jesus Christ? *What does* personal relationship *suggest?* communal relationship *or* fellowship? *How do Paul's words affect your understanding?*

REFLECT

Becoming Ambassadors
2 Corinthians 5:17-21

What does it mean to be in the fellowship of Jesus? It means that we have a distinct identity and unique ways to express that identity. We live striving to imitate Jesus and to do the things that he did. In talking to those difficult Corinthian Christians, Paul made sure that they knew what God was up to in Christ was a work of reconciliation. The world was being reconciled to God.

What's in the Bible?
Read 2 Corinthians 5:17-21. What words or phrases have the most meaning for you in the Bible reading? What thoughts or feelings come to mind when you hear about the "ministry of reconciliation"? about being "ambassadors for Christ"?

Again we hear Paul's confidence. In Christ, God was reconciling the world, so often lost and broken, to the God who had conceived it and borne it in love. Because Christ has done this work, we have a glimpse of how this drama of life is intended to end. Death will not get the last word. All those things that seem beyond redemption or healing will find their wholeness in God. Reconciliation will take place.

Beyond this, though, we are once again invited to participate in what God is up to. It is not just that God has done and will do this. God wants ambassadors for Christ: people who can tell this story and take part in the work of reconciliation. We can help the world mirror in its relationships the relationships within God's beloved community.

So the Corinthians, with all their failures, could become ambassadors for Christ. So we, with all of our reasons for why we are not up to the job, can become reconcilers. This is why there is no small work of reconciliation. Whether the task is helping a small US town welcome refugees or bringing races together in South Africa after years of apartheid, these acts participate in the greater work of God.

> *Where do you have the opportunity to be a reconciler? What divisions grieve you? With whom do you need to be reconciled?*

REFLECT

A Strange and Wonderful Story
1 John 1:1-7

Ultimately we have to ask why the Bible tells us all of these stories about God's invitation into relationship with God and with others. What is it that we learn from hearing about these human people who threw in their lot with God?

What's in the Bible?
Read 1 John 1:1-7. What images or words especially stand out for you in the Bible reading? Why?

REFLECT

It is *all* about relationship. Those who have found their identity in the God of Jesus Christ know that the world is about light and not darkness, about hope and not despair, about community and not isolation. The author of the letter of First John sums it up by saying, "We declare to you what we have seen and heard so that you also may have fellowship with us; and truly our fellowship is with the Father and with his Son Jesus Christ" (1:3).

What the Bible invites us to do is to give ourselves to a strange and wonderful story and to see if it reveals to us something of who we are and to whom we are related. We ourselves are "fearfully and wonderfully made" (Psalm 139:14), and we are uniquely made to seek out our true selves and our purpose in the universe. For centuries communities have found these things in the God of Israel and Jesus Christ and have felt compelled to continue to pass along these stories to generations of subsequent seekers.

How might God be inviting you into the "strange and wonderful story" of relationship with God and one another through Jesus Christ?

REFLECT

The Journey of Listening for God

"What then am I, God? What nature am I? A life powerfully various and manifold and immeasurable."[3] It is no accident that the early church leader Augustine asked this question of God. Having encountered the Bible, he knew that to know himself it was necessary for him to listen within and to listen to God. What Augustine found in his searching was that his life was a mystery and a wonder. He would never finish the journey of listening for God.

You are also a mystery and a wonder. Your life is an ocean that invites you to explore and set sail. The Bible only begins to open up the possibilities that you will discover if you give yourself to this adventure. You will find if you seek the God who moves so stealthily through the pages of the Bible, that you are not only in pursuit of God but also in pursuit of yourself. You may also find that you have new companions, especially if you read the Bible as it is meant to be read—in the company of other travelers.

Here's Why I Care
How have the Bible readings in this chapter changed your understanding of God as one who saves? What difference might this make in your daily life? How can you be "drawn into the story" of God's ongoing restoration and salvation?

A Prayer
God, you surprise us with relationship. You don't leave us alone. You know our hearts, and yet you love us. Help us see ourselves as you see us; in Christ we pray. Amen.

---

[1] Rhodes' son, William Jefferson, is a part-time local pastor in The United Methodist Church, serving on the Eastern Shore of Virginia. He shared some of Ionthe's story with me. Her feat is mentioned in her obituary in the *Virginian-Pilot* newspaper, 10/24/2006. It is also referenced in the article "In This Bond Thriller, He Will Be Swimming the Bay for MDA," by Ted Shockley, in *The Eastern Shore News*, 3/26/1997 (http://www.quantrex.com/stb/STB-news.html).
[2] From *Reading the Old Testament: An Introduction,* by Lawrence Boadt (Paulist Press, 1984); pages 180-81.
[3] From *Confessions*; page 186.

APPENDIX

PRAYING THE BIBLE

Praying the Bible is an ancient process for engaging the Scriptures in order to hear the voice of God. It is also called *lectio divina*, which means "sacred reading." You may wish to use this process in order to become more deeply engaged with the Bible readings offered in each chapter of this study book. Find a quiet place where you will not be interrupted, a place where you can prayerfully read your Bible. Choose a Bible reading from a chapter in this study book. Use the following process to "pray" the Bible reading. After you pray the Bible reading, you may wish to record your experience in writing or through another creative response using art or music.

Be Silent

Open your Bible, and locate the Bible reading you have chosen. After you have found the reading, be still and silently offer all your thoughts, feelings, and hopes to God. Let go of concerns, worries, or agendas. Just *be* for a few minutes.

Read

Read the Bible reading slowly and carefully aloud or silently. Reread it. Be alert to any word, phrase, or image that invites you, intrigues you, confuses you, or makes you want to know more. Wait for this word, phrase, or image to come to you; and try not to rush it.

Reflect

Repeat the word, phrase, or image from the Bible reading to yourself and ruminate over it. Allow this word, phrase, or image to engage your thoughts, feelings, hopes, or memories.

Pray

Pray that God will speak to you through the word, phrase, or image from the Bible reading. Consider how this word, phrase, or image connects with your life and how God is made known to you in it. Listen for God's invitation to you in the Bible reading.

Rest and Listen

Rest silently in the presence of God. Empty your mind. Let your thoughts and feelings move beyond words, phrases, or images. Again, just *be* for a few minutes. Close your time of silent prayer with "Amen"; or you may wish to end your silence with a spoken prayer.